Evidence-Base practice

EVIDENCE-BASE PRACTICE
Clinical Appraisal for Nurses

By

Kenneth E. Anderson

Nicole B. Moose

All Right Reserved

No part of this book may be reproduced, transmitted in any form or by any means electronically, mechanically, photocopying, recording or otherwise without prior permission from the copyright owner.

Evidence-Base practice

Chapter 5..(66)
Critical assessments.

Conclusion..(88)

Evidence-Base practice

CONTENTS

Introduction..(5)

Chapter 1..(7)

What is Evidence-Base practice.

Chapter 2..

Evolution of nursing research.

Chapter 3..

Identifying research questions.

Chapter 4..

Crucial steps in the Evidence-Base pr

Evidence-Base practice

INTRODUCTION

According to the Journal of Nursing Administration, evidence-based practice (EBP) is an approach to healthcare that makes use of the most recent research to improve patients' health and safety, reduce overall costs, and reduce variation in health outcomes. It is applied problem-solving that combines clinical experience, the values and preferences of the patients receiving treatment, and the most recent medical literature's best practices.

Even though EBP only started to become widely used in modern nursing practice in the 1990s, it has a long history in nursing. Although Archie Cochrane, a physician in the 1970s, is credited as the inventor of evidence-based practice (EBP), some nurse researchers attribute it to Florence Nightingale. Her effort to use accurate observation and analysis to improve patient outcomes in the face of unsanitary conditions in the 1800s is frequently regarded as the first instance of EBP.

During the Crimean War, Nightingale used her critical thinking skills, evidence, and experiments to improve patient health at the barrack hospital in Scutari, Turkey. She also used statistics to better predict her patients' mortality and morbidity. She was a pioneer for EBP in nursing, even though she did not have as much research as we do today.

EBP is a natural fit because all nurses have a common heritage that goes back to Nightingale. EBP should be included as an essential component of the curriculum in any online RN to BSN program for nurses. EBP consistently reduces costs, strengthens outcomes, reduces geographic disparities in care, and improves healthcare delivery, according to research. Utilizing EBP has been secured to increment generally speaking position fulfillment, which thus decreases burnout. EBP is becoming the standard of care in the United States slowly, despite its effectiveness in meeting the Triple and Quadruple Aims. It is essential to advance the use of EBP because of its demonstrated capacity to substantially reduce costs while simultaneously enhancing care quality. As members of interdisciplinary teams and healthcare systems, nurses can play an important role in the implementation of EBP if they have the necessary knowledge and skills.

CHAPTER 1

WHAT IS EVIDENCE-BASED PRACTICE (EBP)?

1.1 What Does Evidence-Base Practice Mean? Evidence-based practice (EBP) is the idea that work procedures should be supported by scientific evidence. Even though it seems like a good idea, the idea has been controversial, with some arguing that results might not be as specific to individuals as traditional practices. Since the official introduction of evidence-based medicine in 1992, evidence-based practices have expanded to include allied health professions, education, management, law, public policy, architecture, and other fields. There is also a movement to implement evidence-based practices in scientific research itself in response to studies demonstrating issues in scientific research, such as the replication crisis. Metascience is research into how science is done using evidence.

The trend toward evidence-based practices aims to encourage professionals and other decision-makers to pay more attention to evidence to help them make decisions. In some cases, this may even be a requirement. By shifting the basis for decision making from tradition, intuition, and unsystematic experience to firmly grounded scientific research, evidence-based practice aims to eliminate unsound or outdated practices in favor of

Evidence-Base practice

more effective ones. Clinical decision-making and the application or translation of research findings are examples of evidenced-based practice (EBP).

EBP also involves taking into account the individual requirements and preferences of patients while combining the best evidence with clinical expertise and knowledge. Better patient outcomes are more likely to be achieved when used consistently. When you use EBP, you stop using old ways to give care and choose effective, proven methods to meet the needs of each patient. When using EBP, healthcare professionals need to be able to determine the value of research for their particular patient population.

How to use EBP in clinical practice It would be nearly impossible to evaluate all of the evidence on a subject.

Fortunately, a number of EBP processes have been created to assist health care providers in implementing EBP at work.

Evidence-Base practice

THE SIX STEPS OF THE MOST COMMON PROCEDURE ARE AS FOLLOWS:

1. Make a request. Do you have any questions about the clinical setting in which you work? You might wonder if a new intervention is better than the one you're currently using. Think about it: What is effective and what could be enhanced? And, even more crucially, WHY? Analyze the procedures and workflows that have an effect on the identified practice gap or are affected by it. We'll utilize a configuration called PICO(T) (articulated "pee ko"). The subsequent module covers PICOT questions in greater detail.

2. Obtain the existing evidence. This will be accomplished through a literature search. Your clinical question will direct your search.

3. Examine the sources. Or, in other words, sort, read, and evaluate literature that has been peer reviewed.

4. Make use of your findings when making clinical decisions. Integrate clinical expertise, patient preferences, and values with the evidence. Then, make recommendations for day-to-day practice based on evidence.

5. Evaluate the results. Examine the data and record your strategy. Make sure to include any changes or revisions. Monitor the effects of your intervention closely. Summarize and evaluate the results.

6. The data should be disseminated. Share the project's outcomes with others. Promoting best practices and preventing duplicate work are both aided by sharing. Additionally, it

Evidence-Base practice

enhances the existing resources that either endorse or decry the practice.

Participating in project-based work may teach us how to use EBP, but incorporating it into our daily practice can help us strive for the best patient outcomes. It requires us to consider our practice carefully and ask the appropriate questions.

It is essential to keep in mind that, despite the fact that applying evidence at the bedside can be done independently, working together as a team is more likely to result in long-term improvement.

Before there was evidence... As health care providers, our daily practice ought to prompt inquiries regarding the evidence behind it.

For instance, in the past, neutropenic patients were kept in complete isolation to keep them from getting infections that could kill them. When the best evidence from the study was looked at, it was found that strict isolation precautions did not improve patient outcomes over standard precautions like handwashing, and it appeared that we unnecessarily exposed patients to the negative psychological effects of extreme isolation.

We clinicians frequently adhere to out-of-date policies and procedures without questioning their relevance, accuracy, or the evidence supporting their continued use.

WHAT DIFFERENTIATES EBP FROM RESEARCH?

It is a common misunderstanding that EBP and research are synonymous. Not true! While there are some similarities, their purpose is one of the main differences. The development of new knowledge or the validation of existing knowledge based on a theory is the goal of research. Research includes deliberate, logical request to respond to explicit inquiries or test theories utilizing restrained, thorough strategies. Researchers must use the scientific methods in an orderly, sequential manner in order for their findings to be regarded as reliable and valid. To generate new knowledge or validate existing knowledge based on theory through research and evidence-based practice.   to use the best evidence available to make informed decisions regarding patient care. In contrast, the goal of EBP is to translate the evidence and apply it to clinical practice and decision-making, not to create new

Evidence-Base practice

knowledge or to validate existing knowledge. Utilizing the most up-to-date evidence to make well-informed decisions regarding patient care is the goal of EBP. A large portion of the best proof stems from research, however EBP goes past examination and incorporates the clinical mastery of the clinician and medical services groups, as well as tolerant inclinations and values.

Before you get started, a few important things to keep in mind Research findings should not be used alone to justify a change in practice unless there are other reasons. Other aspects to take into account include:

Values and preferences of the patient Experience of the health care provider Assessment and laboratory results of the patient Data obtained from other sources, such as unit-based metrics and workflow In order for EBP strategies to lead to the best possible outcomes for the patient, each of these aspects needs to be taken into consideration.

We must also consider whether the project will be supported by institutional and administrative resources in order to implement EBP. Take, for instance, the substantial body of research that suggests pregnant women who attend cognitive therapy sessions while they are in the hospital for extended periods of time have lower rates of depression. Even though this is a great idea, it may not be possible to afford to hire a therapist to provide this treatment.

People, or human resources, should come to mind when you think of resources. Who in your company has the ability to help you with the project? Are there key stakeholders or content experts you should involve early

on?

Do you have a strategy for evaluating progress and access to data?

Very much like examination, we should assess and screen any progressions in results subsequent to carrying out an EBP project with the goal that constructive outcomes are upheld and adverse consequences are helped. Even though an intervention may be very effective in a rigorously controlled trial, this does not always mean that it will work exactly the same way for your individual patients or in your clinical setting.

1.2 The evidence hierarchy.

A heuristic used to rank the relative strength of scientific research results is a hierarchy of evidence (or levels of evidence). The relative strength of large-scale epidemiological studies is generally acknowledged. The strength of the evidence is influenced by the design of the study (such as a case report for an individual patient or a blinded randomized controlled trial) and the endpoints

measured (such as survival or quality of life). More than 80 distinct hierarchies have been proposed for evaluating medical evidence. Meta-analyses of randomized controlled trials (RCTs) provide the best evidence for treatment efficacy in clinical research. Systematic reviews of completed, high-quality RCTs, such as those published by the Cochrane Collaboration, rank the same as systematic reviews of completed, high-quality observational studies when it comes to studying side effects. Evidence hierarchies are an essential component of evidence-based medicine (EBM).

The Importance of Nursing Research in Online Programs

Students enrolled in online nursing programs may enroll in research-related courses to enhance their skills. Nursing

Evidence-Base practice

research courses may introduce students to research design and analysis, laying the groundwork for future study of current knowledge. The student will also get an overview of the most recent issues in knowledge development in these classes, which also include evidence-based practice.

The healthcare system of today is complicated, and patients' requirements are changing. Providers with a wide range of perspectives are needed to come up with solutions to the health problems that affect a variety of populations. Online nursing programs may prepare graduates to become professionals who are aware of the significance of nursing research and how to incorporate it into their own practice.

CHAPTER 2

EVOLUTION OF NURSING RESEARCH

The development of a nursing research culture is similar to that of chiropractic in many ways. By looking at key aspects of the evolution of nursing science, there are lessons to be learned and mistakes to be avoided. Since Florence Nightingale in the 19th century, nursing research has undergone significant change. It is evident that nursing research has not always been as influential or significant as it is today. Even after Nightingale's work was published, there was very little research on nursing research. This may be because people have always thought of nursing as an apprenticeship in a task-oriented, caring profession. While research on nursing education and

Evidence-Base practice

administration was done in the first half of the 20th century, nursing research didn't start making the progress it has made over the past three decades until the 1950s.

Numerous factors account for this: the creation of vehicles for the dissemination of nursing research, federal funding and support for nursing research, the enhancement of faculty and student research skills, and an increase in the number of nurses with advanced academic preparation. This article provides a brief overview of the development of nursing research and the theory that has accompanied that development.

Like other practice professions, nursing requires a knowledge foundation that is derived from systematic research and based on theory. Florence Nightingale, the first nursing theorist, was the chief nurse for the British during the Crimean War in the middle of the 1850s. She wrote detailed reports on both medical and nursing matters. That's what songbird noticed "... dread, vulnerability, pausing, assumption, anxiety toward shock, cause a patient more damage than any effort" (p. 6). Consequently, Nightingale's concept of nursing included the requirement for knowledge of natural laws, disease prevention, and personal power use. She emphasized the importance of the patient's environment and the need to care for the patient

Evidence-Base practice

rather than the disease because she saw people as both physical and spiritual beings.

Nutrition, hydration, and sanitation were altered as a result of her emphasis on the environment, and mortality rates significantly decreased during the Crimean War. In ensuing years, Songbird created "laws of nursing" that framed the reason for nursing science and directed nursing training in the US from 1850 to the 1950s.

Teaching was guided by nursing theory rather than research or practice in the 1960s. Nursing's earlier emphasis on education and professional identity naturally led to this. Moreover, the Public Association for Nursing (the expert certifying body) specified a calculated structure for educational plan. The person, the environment, health, and nursing were identified as paradigmatic concepts that are essential to nursing. Scientific efforts were devoted to developing curriculum that corresponded to the current environment at this point, and textbooks emphasized the significance of "holism" in nursing with titles like "The Biopsychosocial Approach." Despite the fact that nurse authors acknowledged the existence of multiple causes in human illness, linear cause-and-effect models rather than multivariate approaches were far too prevalent in research, courses, and textbooks.

Evidence-Base practice

Theories that explained the art and science of nursing emerged in the 1950s and 1960s. Based on her experience as a psychiatric nurse, Hildegard Peplau wrote Interpersonal Relations in Nursing in 1952. Other hypotheses included the 1967 edition of Levine's Conservation Principles of Nursing; Roger published The Science of Unitary Man in 1980, The Science of Unitary Human Beings, a Paradigm for Nursing in 1983, and Roger's Introduction to the Theoretical Basis of Nursing in 1970. A Theory for Nursing was written by Imogene King: Sister Calista Roy published her adaptation model in 1980, and Systems, Concepts, Process was published in 1981. These "grand" theories were difficult to empirically measure, and they were also complicated. Accordingly testing these early nursing speculations through research was troublesome. The recent trend has been to develop and test midrange theories that describe patient problems and nursing practice in light of the emphasis on clinical nursing research.

Evidence-Base practice

NURSING RESEARCH DEVELOPMENT

In 1859, Nightingale used an epidemiological method to describe the morbidity and mortality of sick and injured soldiers in the battlefield hospitals of the Crimean War. Her groundbreaking epidemiological research and statistical methodology, which documented the connection between soldiers' health and the environment, were the hallmarks of nursing's scientific investigation.

Nursing research in the United States was in its infancy from 1900 to 1949, with a focus on nursing education, nurses, nursing students, and ways to organize nurses' work. As was mentioned earlier, nursing theory was only discussed at this time for the purpose of creating and organizing educational curriculum. Early educators were unable to develop educational programs that helped students focus on nursing concepts and problems rather than medical concepts and problems while also representing a nursing perspective. During the first half of this century, groups were established to respond to inquiries like: What exactly is nursing, what are nurses' responsibilities, and how distinct is it from other health science fields? Proficient discussions seethed concerning whether nursing was only a "unfortunate stepsister" of medication or whether it was essential for the natural, normal, or actual sciences. In terms of nursing practice, there was virtually no research conducted during this time.

NURSING: HISTORICAL DEVELOPMENTS IN NURSING THEORY AND RESEARCH

It wasn't until the 1980s that nursing started to focus a lot of its research on patients and how they behave. This was logical because nurses started to see how behavior affects recovery from illness or rehabilitation. When promoting health or preventing illness in the past, nurses acknowledged the contributions of numerous other factors while searching for a single cause. Early on, a culture of nursing research relied heavily on empirical (logical positivist) methods of inquiry. In an effort, perhaps, to seek scientific validation, nurse researchers modeled themselves after colleagues in the basic and biomedical sciences. The use of qualitative research methods like phenomenology and ethnography by nurses to explain complex human phenomena only increased in the 1980s and 1990s. As a result, when the research questions call for a holistic combination of quantitative and qualitative research methodologies, nurse researchers are just beginning to respond to the need to view human problems in terms that are less reductionistic. To improve their comprehension of patient behavior and their capacity to respond constructively to it, many nurses have pursued additional education, consultation, or research over the past two decades. For instance, by the mid-1980s, there was a sizable expansion in nursing investigations of people and families encountering formative, natural, or disease created emergency circumstances including both intense and long haul pressure reactions.

In response to advancements in society, medicine, science, and technology, nursing practice underwent a clinical revolution in the 1990s. As the efforts of individuals within and outside of nursing (such as the National Academy of Science, the National Institute for Nursing Research, and major foundations) coalesced to stimulate and support clinical nursing research, changes in nursing practice began to occur (such as research-based practice guidelines). At the same time, there was a new resurgence of interest among nurses in redefining the issues that arise in their practice and identifying the knowledge gaps that support their practice base. As was mentioned earlier, there has been a lot of interest in qualitative and quantitative research methods for a practice field that has to deal with complicated human phenomena. In the past, descriptive or exploratory research questions were the most frequently addressed by nursing research. However, as they redefine clinical problems and systematically address knowledge gaps, nurse researchers are now going beyond "what is" and "how" questions to address more explanatory or predictive-level questions using methodologically rigorous experimental and quasi-experimental designs. Nursing researchers have grown to include and collaborate on interdisciplinary studies, health care systems and health services research, and taxonomies like the Nursing Intervention Classification (NIC) and Nursing Outcomes Classification (NOC) since they established themselves in the research field. The taxonomies are an attempt to define what nurses do and the outcomes that are responsive to nursing interventions. The culture of nursing research has now advanced to the point where not only research itself but also its application in practice can be taken into account. Research is not the end in and of itself; rather, it is a means by which practice can be improved by utilizing research findings.

Evidence-Base practice

The act of transferring and putting into practice knowledge gleaned from research in order to influence or alter the health care system's current practices is known as research utilization. Summarizing the research-derived knowledge is one of the primary components of research use. distributing the findings of the research to patients, policymakers, nurses, and other health care professionals; and achieving the desired outcomes for patients, their families, and organizations and providers of health care. Beginning with the Western Interstate Commission for Higher Education in Nursing (WCHEN) Regional Program for Nursing Development, models for the utilization of research were developed in the 1970s. Different models remember the Lead and Use of Exploration for Nursing (CURN) project, the Stetler/Marram model, the recovery and use of examination in nursing (RARIN) model, and the Iowa model of exploration practically speaking. Research utilization programs' primary objective is to ensure research-based care delivery models by integrating research findings into nursing practice. Advanced practice nurses can use research utilization as a great example of how to put research findings into practice.

Evidence-based practice, or the use of research findings to guide treatment decisions, is a significant trend. Using this method, a treatment-related question is formulated and the current research's sufficiency is assessed. If the research base is sufficient, protocols are created and implemented, and the evaluation is finished. Through these endeavors, the nursing calling, in organization with different callings, overcomes any barrier among examination and practice to work on quiet consideration.

EDUCATIONAL ADVANCEMENT

Early nursing education was provided through hospital training programs (the nursing diploma), which were modeled after the work that Florence Nightingale did in the United Kingdom. The National League for Nursing (NLN), the educational accrediting body for nursing, called for university-level education in 1915. In 1923, Yale University and Western Reserve University established nursing baccalaureate programs; however, the majority of nursing education was provided through hospital-based diploma programs. The first nursing education programs at a community college opened in 1971, offering associate

degrees in nursing to graduates. Today, associate degree programs are the most common route to nursing practice entry, followed by baccalaureate programs. There are now fewer diploma programs than there were in the past. While nursing students may be introduced to research through associate degree programs, nursing research was included in the upper division curriculum of baccalaureate programs. From 1900 to the 1960s, schools of education provided the majority of nursing leaders with graduate-level training. The Master's degree was regarded as the ultimate nursing degree for many years.

The quantity of attendants whose profession was dedicated to explore was miniscule during the 1960s. In fact, only about 400 nurses in the United States held doctoral degrees by the 1970s. In 1955, the Nursing Exploration Awards and Association Program of the Division of Nursing, US General Wellbeing Administration (USPHS) was laid out. Grants for nursing research projects, fellowships for nursing research, and graduate training for nurse scientists were given out through this program. Because there were no nursing doctoral programs available at the time, the initial funding was for nurses to obtain doctorates in fields other than nursing. Nurse-

anthropologists, nurse-physiologists, and so forth emerged in the field as a result. Although they were educated to conduct research, they frequently remained in their doctoral field and did not apply their research to issues affecting nursing care. The accentuation during this period kept on being on laying out nursing's legitimate spot in the scholarly setting of the college. In many university-based nursing schools, faculty members began to prepare both themselves and their students to become investigators as nursing became more integrated into university life in the 1970s

There are currently three distinct doctoral programs in nursing. The Nursing Doctorate (ND) was first offered at Case Western Reserve University in 1979. It was meant to be the same as a Doctor of Medicine degree, but it did not prepare students for advanced practice or general nursing. Advanced clinical, administrative, or policy-related practice and leadership were emphasized in professional doctorates known as Doctor of Nursing Science (DNS, DNSc, DSN). The Doctor of Nursing Science degree emphasizes practical application and testing of new knowledge rather than basic research. Although the Doctor of Philosophy (PhD) was first offered to nurses at

Teachers College at Columbia University in the 1920s, the 1970s saw a resurgence of interest in doctoral education. Over 65 institutions now offer doctoral programs in nursing, up from zero in the 1950s. Of these, three-quarters are academic doctorates (PhDs), which prepare graduates for a lifetime of research and scholarship. The National Institutes of Health (NIH) has recently provided individual (F32) and institutional (T32) traineeship support to academic nurses interested in pursuing postdoctoral research training.

Support and funding for research During the 1980s and 1990s, a number of factors contributed to the expansion of nursing research. The establishment of the National Center for Nursing Research (NCNR) within the United States Public Health Service (USPHS) in 1986 may have been the most significant factor. The American Nurses' Association (ANA) took strong political action, which led to the establishment of this Center. "the conduct, support, and dissemination of information regarding basic and clinical nursing research, training, and other programs in patient care research" was the NCNR's primary objective (p. 2). Prior to the NCNR's establishment, the majority of federal funding for research was allocated to medical

studies focusing on disease diagnosis and treatment. Thus, the establishment of the NCNR was a significant accomplishment for nurse researchers. The NCNR changed its name to the National Institute of Nursing Research (NINR) in 1993, giving the Center institute status within the NIH and bolstering nursing's position. As a result of this development, nursing was elevated to a position of greater equality with scientists and other health professions in the mainstream of research activities. With the foundation of the Middle and afterward the Organization, government subsidizing for nursing research has developed. The NCNR had a budget of $16.2 million in 1986. The NINR had a budget of approximately $55 million in 1996, more than tripling in a decade. The NINR decided to support the following five areas of research from 1995 to 1999: models of community nursing, the efficacy of HIV/AIDS nursing interventions, cognitive impairment, living with chronic illness, and immunocompetence-related biobehavioral factors.

The funding of nursing research on chronic diseases (such as improving adherence to chemotherapy and pain relief), quality and cost-effectiveness of care, health promotion and disease prevention, management of symptoms (such as gender differences in response to therapeutics and managing the pain cycle), health disparities (such as cultural sensitivity), adaptation to new technologies (such as transplants), and palliative care at the end of life are all included in the NINR's strategic plan for the next millennium. Although investigator-initiated research topics are funded if they are significant to nursing or patient care, special allocations and RFAs have facilitated research in these target areas. Over $70 million is anticipated for NINR's budget for the year 2000, which is roughly divided as follows: 73 percent for grants for outside research projects; 8% for training before and after a doctorate; 3.5% for profession advancement; 3.5 percent for Core Centers in specialized research areas; 3% to go toward the intramural program. The NINR and the scientific community welcome the challenge of planning research for the next five years and a century.

DISSEMINATION OF RESEARCH

Significant junctures in the growth of nursing science began in the middle of the 1950s. Between the years 1950 and 1959, there was a growing emphasis on the need to

find a body of knowledge for the growing nursing profession in order to justify its presence in universities after World War II. Not exclusively was the principal diary of Nursing Exploration laid out in 1952; Additionally, a number of nursing research-related textbooks were published. The American Nurses Association established the American Nurses Foundation specifically to promote nursing research, which was another significant step in the development of the culture of nursing science. Regional research conferences were first established in the 1950s, and federal funding for nursing research began. The development of a nursing science relied on all of these factors.

Evidence-Base practice

At the end of the 1980s, a number of new nursing research journals were established, one of which was Applied Nursing Research (ANR). The ANR publishes research papers that are particularly important to nurse clinicians. Data-based articles are increasingly appearing in clinical specialty journals like Heart and Lung and Journal of Gerontological Nursing. One more significant occasion in the turn of events and dispersal of nursing hypothesis and exploration was the production of the Yearly Survey of Nursing Exploration in 1983. Nursing practice, nursing

care delivery, nursing education, and the nursing profession are all covered in this publication's critical analyses of relevant research. Chapters assess nursing knowledge development in a systematic manner, encourage the application of research findings in practice, and offer guidance for future research. The Encyclopedia of Nursing Research, a publication that provides a comprehensive overview of research studies, the history of nursing research, and the development of nursing theory, was created more recently by scholars.

CHAPTER 3

IDENTIFYING RESEARCH QUESTIONS

4.1 Developing research Questions

A research project begins with an idea that is then transformed into a research question. Identifying research questions Creating a research question Observations made by health care workers in the NHS lead to a lot of research questions that could help patients. These include improved approaches to service organization and delivery as well as potential clinical innovations.

Evidence-Base practice

A research question is a statement that describes the research's goals and potential outcomes in clear, focused, and concise terms. It should drive the creation of a research protocol because it determines the success of a research procedure. The language used to express a research question should be straightforward and easy to understand.

Research questions can be derived from a variety of sources, including peer conversations, clinical practice, the scientific literature, and quality improvement activities. There are a variety of useful methods, like mind mapping, brainstorming, and focus groups, that can be used to develop and refine research ideas.

The PICOT format is a very helpful method for converting a research idea into a research question. P is a mnemonic for the terms "population," "intervention," "comparison," "outcome," and "timeframe." The population is the sample of participants who will be recruited for the study. It is critical to indicate the attributes of the qualified members like age, orientation, identity, social class, disease(s), the enrollment setting and so on. This also requires defining who would be excluded (for instance, patients with particular conditions). The treatment or activity that will be provided to the study's participants is referred to as the "intervention." Consider the dose, duration,

Evidence-Base practice

frequency, intensity, timing, route, intervention administrator, and other factors. In some studies, a disease, physical condition, accessibility issue, or organizational issue may take the place of intervention.

C refers to the reference that you intend to compare with the treatment. In the event that there is a current 'highest quality level' treatment, you ought to expect to involve it as a correlation. A correlation can be inert or dynamic, fake treatment, no treatment, regular consideration, an alternate variation of a similar intercession, an elective mediation and so forth.

O: The outcome is the thing that will be measured to see how well the intervention worked. It is essential to consider the type of outcome (such as showing benefit or harm, clinical events or patient-reported outcomes, dichotomous or continuous, etc.), the method by which the outcomes will be measured, the time at which they will be measured, etc. The validity, relevance, and applicability of the findings may be impacted by the study's length, frequency of measurements, and time.

Questions about what, how, and why are another useful method for coming up with a research question:

What is the purpose of this study? The purpose of this question is to ascertain the objectives and rationale of the research.

What will the research reveal about the answer to your inquiry? The focus of this question is on figuring out the best research design and method to answer the research question.

Why is it important to respond to this research question? Given that conducting research involves investing time, effort, money, and other resources, the purpose of this question is to provide justification for doing so.

The FINER acronym, which stands for feasible, interesting, novel, ethical, and relevant research question, encapsulates the characteristics of a good research question.

Evidence-Base practice

The study's feasibility includes the practical aspects of conducting research. To get a clear understanding of how the project will be carried out, it is essential to consider the

project's feasibility. It's critical to find out if the question can be answered in a particular setting and within a predetermined, attainable time frame. To carry out the study, researchers ought to take into consideration the requirements for facilities, tools, expertise, and training. When you think about these things, you can better understand what kind of additional support is needed and where it can be found.

It is necessary to explain why a research question matters, such as to patient outcomes, and what the subsequent benefit will be in order to demonstrate that it is interesting. Specialists ought to introduce the size, seriousness and the weight of the issue they need to address or likely effect on assistance or populace and exhibit that the exploration is required in view of the hole in the information and proof.

A literature review is required to ensure that the research question is novel and has not already been investigated. Please read Systematic reviews to support primary research applications in the Resources section of this website for additional guidance. In addition, improving the research question and selecting the best methodology may benefit from a literature review. New information

should come from research projects. However, research studies may also be replicated when their design or analysis flaws make their findings unreliable.

It is necessary to guarantee the ethical conduct of the research study. It's important to think about things like informed consent, privacy, confidentiality, and anonymity, ownership of data, conclusions, and how to use and misuse results, and other things like that. Additionally, researchers should consider minimizing patient discomfort and safeguarding limited resources. Additionally, it is important to take into consideration the particular ethical concerns that are associated with particular patient groups, such as adults or children with dementia. Also, researchers should try to figure out why people might stop participating in the intervention studies and how the negative effects will be recorded.

The demonstration of the relevance of the research question is yet another crucial step. The applied wellbeing research, which is qualified for NIHR subsidizing, should add to further developed medical care practice and give clear patients benefits.

Evidence-Base practice

Making a question that can be researched: A crucial step in facilitating good clinical research One of the challenging tasks a researcher faces when starting a project is coming up with a researchable question. An investigator may initiate the formulation of a clinical research question in response to either unanswered issues in current clinical practice or when experiences dictate the use of alternative therapies. By providing step-by-step instructions for formulating a research question, this article will be of assistance to researchers. In addition, the PICO (population, intervention, control, and outcomes) criteria for framing a research question are described in this paper.

An uncertainty about a problem that can be challenged, examined, and analyzed to provide useful information is referred to as a "researchable question." How well an investigator formulates the research question based on the issues encountered in day-to-day research activities and clinical practice is critical to the success of a project. A significant amount of information can be gleaned from a research project's underlying questions regarding the topic's relevance, researchability, and significance. A well-formulated research question necessitates extreme specificity and precision, which guides the project's

implementation in light of the identification of the population and variables of interest. In this section, a clinical scenario will be presented, and we will observe how clinical questions arise and assist us in locating evidence to answer our question.

CASE: A 2-year-old boy comes into an outpatient clinic with a fever and severe pain in his right ear. This is how the research question is formulated. His mother is concerned about the fact that he has been taking the antibiotic amoxicillin for the past few weeks because he has a history of having recurring ear infections. She is concerned about the long-term effects of taking antibiotics. Additionally, she is concerned about the outcome of recurring ear infections. She wants to know if the antibiotic amoxicillin is effective or if it can be replaced due to its side effects, like frequent diarrhea.

This case raises a number of questions that can be broadly divided into background and foreground questions. "Background Questions" are general questions about a disease or clinical problem. These inquiries typically inquire about the disease, disorder, or treatment in terms of what, when, how, and where, such as "What is otitis media?" or "What is the action of ampicillin?" etc. Reading review articles or textbooks can provide answers to these kinds of questions.

"Foreground Questions" are patient-oriented inquiries that consider risk versus benefit for a patient or group of patients and involve interpretation of a therapy or disease. Primary or pre-assessed studies in the literature are the best sources of information for these kinds of difficult clinical questions. The majority of these questions compare two things, such as two diagnostic techniques, treatments, or drugs.

For framing a "foreground" research question, the PICO (population, intervention, control, and outcomes) format is thought to be a well-known method. Sackett and co pointed out that breaking the question into its four parts will make it easier to find relevant data.

Problem or population: focusing on a particular population, its most important characteristics, and demographic data. From the above case, you can recognize pediatric populace with otitis media, the age range, sex, introducing grievance, and history.

Evidence-Base practice

The intervention can be a procedure, diagnostic test, treatment, or treatment of interest, as well as risk or prognostic factors. In this instance, the plan you have for treating the patient will be the intervention, which could be a new treatment, a diagnostic test, a prognostic factor, or a procedure. For instance, based on your observations in the clinic, cefuroxime is a more effective treatment option for otitis media than amoxicillin, but you are uncertain about its efficacy in children with otitis media.

When a new therapy is contrasted with an existing one, it is called a comparator or control.

The outcome is what the intervention did. Take, for instance, how well it manages pain. As a result, the patient's condition may improve, the infection may be eradicated, or the risk of developing resistance may be reduced. A good primary outcome should be relevant to your research question, easily quantifiable, specific, valid, and reproducible. A clinician must be familiar with both background and foreground questions in a typical clinical setting, depending on their prior knowledge of a particular disease and its treatment. Complexer questions are addressed after background questions are answered. The central issues in a clinical work are the source of the

clinical questions. Examples include etiological questions about causes or risk factors, diagnostic queries about sensitivity and

Evidence-Base practice

specificity, therapeutic questions about the best treatment options, and prognostic questions about the treatment's outcome.

The PICO method is used once a foreground question has been selected. The question is easier to search when broken down into parts. In this instance, there are a number of pertinent questions, such as: What are the outcomes of having an ear infection that comes back, what might happen if antibiotics are used for a long time, and what are the side effects of the current treatment? The following researchable questions can be formulated if all of the information from the PICO approach is gathered.

Is cefuroxime (I) more effective than amoxicillin (C) at shortening the duration of symptoms in children with acute otitis media (P)?

Will children with otitis media receive an improvement in symptoms and a decrease in the likelihood of developing resistance to cefuroxime?

Children with otitis media treated with amoxicillin face an increased risk of developing resistance.

Is surgery better for treating otitis media in children than using antibiotics over and over again?

Based on our patient's illness and concerns, we have formulated multiple questions from the preceding case. We can now employ the method of "selecting" the best question. For instance, which inquiry is more significant to the well-being of the patient, which inquiry is pertinent to our knowledge requirements, and which inquiry may provide intriguing responses to our patients' and clinical inquiries? In addition, we need to think about whether or not it would be possible to locate the evidence quickly.

Surveying The Exploration Questions With Regards to A Review Plan

As proposed by Hulley et al. The FINER (feasible, interesting, novel, ethical, and relevant) criteria should be considered when formulating a research question, and the response should fill in any knowledge gaps. When evaluating a research question, the following factors should be taken into consideration.

The feasibility of a research project is based on the research question and should be considered early in the process to avoid wasting resources and intellectual energy. Determining the required resources A novice investigator needs guidance from their mentors because this can be challenging for them at times.

To determine whether it is possible, you might want to conduct a pilot or proof-of-concept study;

Early on in the project, consult a biostatistician to select a less expensive design and common outcomes;

Consider the possibility of enrolling the desired number of subjects from your interest's population. Also, if it's hard to enroll the intended number of people, think about expanding your inclusion criteria and changing your exclusion criteria; and think about how much each part of the study's design, research team, and resources will cost.

Relevance and significance of making it interesting An important question may not appear interesting in its presentation. It is difficult to clearly present a research question and attract reviewers' interest and attention. It's too much work to not be passionate about the subject of your research. If the subject is novel and also piques the

interest of your collaborators, coworkers, and the community as a whole, you will receive more support for your research and will find it simpler to publish. It is essential to pursue a research question with a burning desire to uncover the truth. This is how everyone views research; commitment to a high-quality, unbiased, and systematic project completion. Your project can get a lot of support if your question can explain a problem and point to a specific aspect that is missing.

CONDUCTING A LITERATURE REVIEW

A comprehensive literature search determines the innovation of any research question. As it stands, there is no need to repeat the study in any way that is already documented in the literature. If your question approaches an existing problem in a novel way, depending on the research question, the study may be replicated. This can be accomplished by connecting two distinct studies whose outcomes did not resolve the issue or by employing distinct populations, new conceptual approaches, or innovative techniques. A literature search should be conducted after a preliminary question has been

formulated to determine what is known and unknown about the subject. The purpose of the literature review is to find out what research has been done on the subject of interest. how exactly has it been carried out? also, what are the knowledge gaps? PubMed, MedlinePlus, CINAHL, or Web of Science are the primary search databases that should be used, but other databases can also be used. PubMed clinical query is a user-friendly database for searching for clinical practice-related evidence. In addition, this provides information for performing categorical searches in MEDLINE, such as therapeutic, diagnostic, etiological, and prognostic. For finding evidence on therapeutic issues, the American College of Physicians (ACP) and clinical evidence from BMJ Publishing Group are excellent sources. Other search engines, like OVID, offer access to other databases, like the Cochrane Library, where full-text articles and systematic reviews can be found. These databases include a large selection of books and journals. Gray and co. suggested 4 Ss for a review of the literature: Systems: making use of all available resources, Synopses: obtaining high-quality study abstracts and synopses, studies, systematic reviews: original studies of research Systematic reviews are regarded as the most effective method for gathering

evidence in the hierarchy of evidence-based medicine. Systematic reviews are rigorous approaches to combining the findings of numerous high-quality studies. Since we want to find a difference, conducting a thorough literature search also helps us determine the sample size, the methodology, and the type of analysis. A new study's structure and the scientific community's knowledge gaps can only be filled with this information.

Step by step instructions to explain a clinical inquiry

Clinical inquiries emerge persistently in day to day clinical practice. It is essential that these questions be answered using evidence. A crucial first step toward providing an answer that will guide a decision or allow a researcher to frame the research that will be conducted is to clarify the key aspects of the question.

A well-thought-out question is more likely to result in a trustworthy and useful response, whereas a poorly formulated question can result in ambiguity and confusion. The population and the intervention should be specific, but

keep in mind that it may be difficult to locate relevant studies or sufficient data to provide a reliable response if either or both are described too narrowly. For the populace, this could allude to individuals with an ailment, or in danger of sickness, and determining phase of illness or clinical context might be significant. Diagnostic or screening tests to therapeutic interventions of any kind are examples of interventions. It may be necessary to provide a thorough explanation of the intervention and comparator, such as the method of administration, dosage, treatment duration, or the various components of a complex intervention. Alternative competing interventions, variations of standard care, or no treatment or a placebo could serve as the most appropriate comparator. Surrogate outcomes, such as bone density, should not typically be taken into consideration unless they can be shown to be directly linked to patient important outcomes. The outcomes that should be considered should be those that are thought to be the most important to patients or other decision makers. A logic framework is frequently essential for elucidating potential action paths in complex questions.

A credible answer can be found by clarifying a good question; however, the certainty of the answer is another important issue to address. Using the GRADE method to evaluate certainty (or the quality of a body of evidence) is essential to this end. Any research question needs to take this into account right away. The initial step comprises of featuring those PICO components, and specifically examinations and results that are basic for independent direction and separating these from those that are significant yet not basic and those that are not significant. In addition, it will be helpful to pre-determine what constitutes a minimum important difference or effect for many outcomes in order to assist in the interpretation of the analysis's findings and guide decision-making.

The nature of the studies that contribute data to the answer to the question is an important part of the GRADE approach. In most cases, the randomised controlled trial is still the most trustworthy method for determining therapeutic interventions' effectiveness. Consequently, the GRADE method initially views RCTs as providing high-quality evidence and observational studies as providing low-quality evidence. This evidence rating may then be decreased or increased (for non-randomized studies)

based on a variety of factors (lower: design flaws, inconsistentness, indirectness, impreciseness, or publication bias, as well as: large effect, dose response, and potential for confounding factors). How we use the data obtained in response to our question will be determined by the final GRADE rating of the evidence for each outcome, which ranges from high, where we are extremely confident that the real effect lies close to the effect estimate, to very low, where we are extremely uncertain about the estimate. Designing a well-thought-out question is essential for obtaining trustworthy responses in a world where health data are becoming increasingly accessible. However, since data are increasingly coming from a variety of different and multiple sources (such as regulatory agency databases and repositories rather than scientific journals, wearable devices, smartphone apps, and social networking sites), creating a clear and focused question may only be the first step in a complicated chain of events that eventually leads to the desired result. While it will be necessary in the not-too-distant future to develop new techniques for combining and synthesizing information from a variety of sources, making effective use of the resources at hand may assist in directing the day-to-day work of clinicians.

CHAPTER 4

CRUCIAL STEPS IN THE EVIDENCE-BASED PRACTICE PROCESS

This is the critical appraisal of evidence to comprehend best practice.

You can ensure that you have the best evidence to treat your patient by evaluating the studies you find in your database searches.

A clinician can use appraisal tools to evaluate evidence for its validity, dependability, and suitability for clinical practice. An article is evaluated using an appraisal tool for the following factors:

The following is a list of critical appraisal tools that are utilized in evidence-based medicine:

Relevance to your clinical question Relevance of the research question being answered Legitimacy of the conclusions Any potential conflicts of interest.

Consensus-based standards for selecting health measurement instruments (COSMIN) are a set of guidelines for assessing the methodological quality of studies on the properties of health measurement instruments.

Evidence-Base practice

Checklists for eight different types of research, including systematic reviews, qualitative studies, randomized controlled trials, case control studies, and diagnostic studies, are available from the Critical Appraisal Skills Program (CASP). There are yes/no and open-ended questions on each checklist.

Josephine Briggs: Basic Examination Instruments

JBI produces 13 apparatuses used to evaluate various investigations or levels of proof. An overall evaluation decision is at the end of each checklist, which includes a series of critical appraisal questions.

The questions in the Johns Hopkins Research Evidence Appraisal Tool make it easier to evaluate an article's study design and evidence level. This tool uses either a 16-item checklist for research studies or a 12-item checklist for systematic reviews and meta-analyses and has three questions that help the reviewer figure out how a study was done.

A tool for evaluating systematic reviews of randomized controlled trials is the **AMSTAR** measurement tool. **AMSTAR 2** can be used to evaluate non-randomised systematic reviews.

Newcastle-Ottawa scale (NOS)

Evidence-Base practice

A device for evaluating and surveying non-randomized examinations remembered for a meta-investigation.

Critical evaluation tools for systematic reviews, randomized controlled trials, and diagnostic and prognostic studies from the Oxford Centre for Evidence-Based Medicine (CEBM).

QUADAS-2

An instrument for surveying the nature of indicative precision studies.

ROBINS-I Bias in Intervention Studies that Aren't Randomized examines the possibility of bias in studies comparing the effects of two or more interventions on health.

Cochrane's risk of bias tool for randomized trials is the RoB2.0 tool.

Fortifying the Announcing of Observational Examinations in The study of disease transmission (STROBE)

Assessment agendas for companion, case-control and cross-sectional examinations.

The next thing you should do after finding some research studies that might help your practice is to critically examine those studies to find the best evidence so that your practice is based on the best information that is available. Research evidence, clinical expertise, and patients' choices and concerns are the best elements of evidence to incorporate into decision-making for evidence-informed nursing practice (Wilkins, 2013). A systematic approach to assessing a research study's strengths and weaknesses, as well as its practical applicability, is known as critical appraisal. "It's in a journal," is a prevalent assumption. Isn't that sufficient? The response is "No,

really not." Even if a paper is published in a peer-reviewed journal, it does not guarantee its quality or clinical relevance. How can you tell if a research study was carried out correctly and whether the data are trustworthy and applicable to your practice? When research on the same subject yields contradictory results, how can you make a decision about what to believe? Critical appraisal skills can be helpful in this situation.

Critical evaluation might sound intimidating. However, you do this occasionally each day. Whether you are perusing the paper, utilizing virtual entertainment or sitting in front of the TV, you process what you read, see, and learn through your encounters. You are savvy consumers of information, filtering it to concentrate on the essentials. You scrutinize the assertions made; You don't take anything for granted. You really want to

Evidence-Base practice

do exactly the same thing when you fundamentally evaluate research studies.

What exactly are you evaluating critically? You are evaluating a research study's quality and determining whether or not the findings can be used in your own clinical situation. When conducting a critical evaluation, the three primary inquiries to answer are:

★ Are the study's findings reliable?
★ What were the outcomes?
★ Will the findings assist me in taking care of my patients?

The validity of the study's findings is the subject of the first inquiry: Did the researcher make use of the most effective approaches to collect the data? Validity is important because oncology nurses need to be able to trust the conclusions drawn by researchers if they want research to help them in their work. When rigorous methods have been used in the research, it is believable and credible. The jargon used to describe research methods can be confusing to many nurses, making critical appraisal even more daunting. Counsel a glossary of normal examination phrasing when you see a new word. Any introductory research textbook or the Internet (such as the Centre for Evidence-Based Medicine) contains a glossary of common research terms.

Evidence-Base practice

The subsequent inquiry tends to the aftereffects of the review — are the outcomes measurably huge or could they have happened by some coincidence? If oncology nurses implemented the intervention in their own practices, would similar outcomes be anticipated? To evaluate the results, you do not need to be an expert statistician; You only need to be able to comprehend the clinical significance of a statistical test. If you need an explanation for a statistical test with which you are unfamiliar, you can look it up in any textbook on introductory statistics or ask a question in the CANO/ACIO online community using the Sosido Network.

The third question inquires about the study's applicability to your area of practice—were the findings found in a population that was comparable to my patients? Do the advantages outweigh the disadvantages? This question is important because it's easy to get caught up in the specifics of the research's methods and outcomes and forget how they apply to actual patients.

How do I respond to these inquiries? To evaluate a research study, I recommend making use of a rapid critical appraisal checklist like the Critical Appraisal Skills Programme (CASP) checklists. You can download these checklists for free. Plunk down with the exploration study and agenda, and work through the inquiries on the agenda. The majority of checklists will include specific subquestions about what constitutes a well-conducted research study for the research design you are evaluating

(e.g., qualitative study, randomized control trial). You probably won't have the option to respond to a portion of the inquiries on the agenda, which is okay. A useful evaluation of the study will begin to emerge if you simply examine it in the most objective way possible. Keep in mind that there is no flawless research study; Every study has its limitations. You will be better able to distinguish studies with minor limitations that can still be used to inform practice (especially when viewed in the context of other research studies) from studies that provide no useful information as you become more familiar with the process.

You can improve your critical appraisal skills in a few ways. In a group setting, journal clubs are a good way to practice critical appraisal. A journal club is a group of people who regularly meet in person or online to evaluate research studies critically. Through this cooperative exertion, you can work on how you might interpret research strategies and keep educated regarding advancements applicable to your training.

Evidence-Base practice

Reading pre-appraised sources is yet another method for raising your level of proficiency. When conducting a critical evaluation of a study, using pre-appraised sources can

help you identify the questions that you ought to be asking. Examples of pre-appraised sources of evidence on a clinical topic include evidence summaries found in library databases, such as Evidence-Based Care Sheets in CINAHL. These summaries are typically prepared by experts and are intended for use at the point of care. Journals that take research that has been published elsewhere, summarize it, and offer expert commentary on it (such as Evidence-Based Nursing) are another pre-appraised source of evidence.

A number of McMaster University's free online learning modules, developed by the National Collaborating Centre for Methods and Tools (NCCMT), can also help you improve your critical appraisal abilities. Interactive online activities to practice critical appraisal skills are included in the modules. Even though these modules are focused on public health, the critical appraisal skills you learn can be used in oncology nursing or any other health care field. You can complete the modules on your own or with a group. You can complete the NCCMT modules at your own pace; You can log in whenever it's convenient for you, pause whenever it's necessary, and resume where you left off. For each module, you can also get a certificate of

completion that you can put in your portfolio. A significant message to detract from perusing this Exploration Reflections segment is that basic examination is an expertise you can create with training. You are not supposed to have a deep understanding of basic examination. In order to carry out critical evaluation in a meaningful manner, you do not need to be an expert in statistics or research. You only need to be able to locate the resources necessary to conduct the critical evaluation and discuss the results with coworkers.

Critical evaluation of clinical research Decisions regarding patient value and care are carefully made by integrating the best available evidence, clinical experience, and patient preference in an essential process. The process of carefully and methodically examining research to determine its validity, value, and relevance for professionals' crucial clinical decision-making is known as critical appraisal.

Basic examination is fundamental to:

Combat excessive information;

Find papers that have a clinical significance;

CPD stands for continuing professional development.

Conducting a Critical Evaluation:

A crucial step in critical evaluation of the study is evaluating the research methods used. Checklists that are specific to the study design are used to accomplish this.

Commonly Asked Questions:

1. What is the purpose of the study?
2. What is the design (type) of the study?

Issues with selection.

- What are the result factors and how are they estimated?
- How are the factors of the study measured, and what are they?

Evidence-Base practice

- What significant potential confounders are thought of?
- What is the study's statistical approach?

Results from statistics.

➢ Concerning the research question, what conclusions did the authors arrive at?

➢ Are moral issues taken into account?

Evidence-Base practice

CHAPTER 5

THE CRITICAL ASSESSMENT BEGINS WITH A REVIEW OF THE FOLLOWING PRIMARY SECTIONS:

I. A Quick Look at the Paper:

The year and publication journal The title of the article: Does it specify important trial goals?

The author(s) and their institution(s) The inclusion of a peer review procedure in journal acceptance protocols also strengthens the evaluation criteria for research papers and reduces the likelihood of low-quality research being published. Author declarations of interest and the possibility of market bias should also be taken into

consideration. To check for a conflict of interest, pay close attention to any declared funding or the issue of a research grant.

II. ABSTRACT:
A quick way to learn about the article's purpose, major procedures and methods, major findings, and conclusions is to read the abstract.

The study's objective: It should be written well and clearly.

Methods and Materials: It should be clear that the study's design, groups, randomization method, sample size, gender, age, and procedure for each group, as well as the measuring instrument(s), were mentioned.

Results: The variables that were measured, their statistical significance and analysis.

Conclusion: It must provide a clear response to the relevant inquiry.

III. Section of introduction and background:

An excellent introduction will make extensive use of references to earlier work that is related to the subject at hand and explain the significance and drawbacks of what has already been acknowledged.

Why is this investigation deemed necessary? What is the study's purpose? Was the purpose established prior to the study, or was a random result discovered during "data searching"?

What has already been accomplished and how does this study differ from previous ones?

-Does the scientific approach outline the intervention or observation's potential benefits and potential drawbacks?

IV. Techniques and Materials area:
All relevant info on how the review was really done ought to be referenced. Exact data is given on the review plan, the populace, the example size and the intercessions introduced. It is important to clearly state each method of measurement.

V. Section of Results:
What actually happens to the subjects should be made abundantly clear in this section. The outcomes could contain crude information and make sense of the factual investigation. Related tables, graphs, and diagrams can show these.

VI. Section for discussion: The clinical relevance of what has recently been established and what has already been identified ought to be completely compared in this section. A conversation on a potential related constraints and necessitation for additional examinations ought to likewise be demonstrated.

- ❖ Does it provide a summary of the study's main findings and link them to any issues with the study's design or execution? Intention to treat analysis is the term for this).

- ❖ Does it address any potential sources of bias?
- ❖ Are the results consistent with the interpretations?

- ❖ How should null results be interpreted?
- ❖ Does it explain how this study's findings relate to previous research in the field?
- ❖ Can they be applied to all situations (external validity)?
- ❖ Is their clinical relevance or applicability mentioned?
- ❖ How applicable are the findings, outcomes, and results to a clinical practice?
- ❖ Does the study's question get answered in the conclusion?

- ❖ Does the conclusion hold up?
- ❖ Is the paper ethically acceptable?
- ❖ Can you think of any possible ethical problems?
- ❖ Are the findings applicable to the population in question?
- ❖ Will you make use of the study's findings?

Whenever you have addressed the fundamental and key inquiries and recognized the exploration strategy utilized, you can integrate explicit inquiries connected with every technique into your evaluation cycle or agenda.

1-What is the purpose of the study?

A study must address a significant healthcare issue and produce novel or significant findings in order to be valuable. The Problem Intervention Comparison Outcome

(PICO) method is a useful structure for evaluating the issue discussed in the article.

P = Patient or issue: Patient/Problem/Population:

It entails determining whether the research has a specific question. What is the main issue?

E.g.,: Status of the disease, previous conditions, medications taken, etc.,

Intervention, I mean: Clearly and appropriately stated management strategy, such as: new procedures, treatments, and diagnostic tests,

Comparison: C = A substitute or appropriate control, such as: specific and restricted to a single option.

O= Results: It is necessary to identify the desired outcomes or patient-related consequences. e.g.,: reducing

symptoms, enhancing performance, enhancing appearance, etc.,

The best study designs are determined by the clinical question.

2-What is the design (type) of the study?

The study's usefulness is fundamentally dependent on its design. In a clinical paper, the method used to get the results is explained in detail. In general, all inquiries regarding the related clinical question, the study design, the subjects, and the correlated measures to reduce bias and confounding ought to be adequately and thoroughly investigated and answered.

Participants and the Sample:

The population of interest to researchers is determined. As a result, a sample population is taken, and the findings from this sample are applied to the target population.

The sample should be accurate representations of the intended audience. It is important to know the sample population's baseline characteristics because this lets researchers see how closely the subjects match their own patients.

Power calculation and sample size calculation: If a beneficial effect exists, a trial should be large enough to have a high detection rate. Analysts can figure out before the preliminary starts how huge the example size ought to be to have a decent possibility distinguishing a genuine contrast between the intercession and control gatherings.

Evidence-Base practice

Is there a defined sample? Animals (types) and humans; Which group of people does it belong to?

Does it provide reasons for the eligibility criteria?

Is it clear where and how the sample was selected, recruited, and evaluated?

Does it specify the location of the study?

Is the size of the sample necessary? Exactly as planned? Is it sufficient to identify clinically and statistically significant outcomes?

Is a suitable study design or type mentioned?

Is the type of study suitable for the research question?

Is the concentrate enough controlled? Is the kind of randomization process mentioned? Does it provide an explanation for or mention the absence of a control group?

Are the examples comparable at pattern? Does sample attrition come up?

At the beginning of each study, the number of participants or specimens is reported, along with details about how many of them completed the study and any reasons for incomplete follow-up.

Which person was blinded is mentioned? Are the participants and assessors aware of the received interventions?

Is the method of data analysis mentioned?

Is it likely that any measurements taken are accurate?

Instruments and methods for measuring have been shown to be accurate and reliable by researchers.

The degree to which a test measures what it is supposed to measure is referred to as validity.

(The degree to which the obtained value accurately reflects the object of interest.)

-The accuracy and soundness of the measuring instrument;

-What is the test's objective?

-Is it measuring precisely what it is intended to measure?

-How effectively and precisely does it measure?

Reliability: In research, reliability refers to a test's repeatability or consistency. Reliability measures a test's consistency across multiple measurements. It is significant especially if tests are given at different times or by different people. Studies ought to express the strategy for surveying the dependability of any estimations taken and what the intra-analyst unwavering quality was.

Issues with selection:

The following inquiries ought to be asked:

- How were participants selected or recruited? In the event that not irregular, would they say they are illustrative of the populace?

- Are Single, Double, or Triple Blinding (Masking) Types Available?

- Does a control group exist? Which one was chosen?

- How do patients get follow-up care? Who are those who drop out? Why are there so many?

- Are the study's independent (predictor) and dependent (outcome) variables well-defined, measured, and clearly identified?

Evidence-Base practice

- Is there a statement regarding issues with sample size or statistical power, which are particularly significant in negative studies?

- If a multicenter study, what quality confirmation measures were utilized to get consistency across destinations?

- Do selection biases exist?

• For a situation control study, in the event that exercise propensities to be looked at:

- Are the controls useful?

- Were the case and control records independently examined?

- How were potential selection biases, such as preponderance bias, admission rate bias, volunteer bias, recall bias, lead time bias, detection bias, and so on, controlled?

Intersectional Research:

- Was the sample chosen correctly (randomly, for convenience, etc.)?

- Were endeavors made to guarantee a decent reaction rate or to limit the event of missing information?

Evidence-Base practice

- Were validity and reliability (reproducibility) reported?

• How were subjects recruited and assigned to groups in an intervention study?

• How many people in a cohort study completed the final follow-up?

- Are the subject's agents of the populace to which the discoveries are applied?

- Is volunteer bias a possibility? Was there enough time for follow-up?

- How many students dropped out?

- The results may not accurately reflect the truth if the methodology is flawed. Patients could suffer harm if these results are used to alter clinical practice.

Matching, restriction, randomization, and blinding are just a few of the methods used by researchers to strengthen the approach.

An error that was not caused by chance at any stage of the study is known as bias. Results that are systematic deviations from the truth are the result of bias. To reduce bias, researchers must rely on effective research design because bias cannot be measured. A study's sample population should be representative of the general population to avoid bias. The study's sample size must also be taken into consideration, as must the study's

power to produce statistically significant results (p-values quoted below 0.05).

4-How are the outcome factors measured and defined?

-Have all pertinent outcomes been evaluated?

-Does measurement error play a significant role in bias?

5-How are the factors of the study measured?

-The study includes all relevant study factors.

-Have the appropriate instruments been used to measure the factors?

Results and Analysis:

It is necessary to evaluate the statistical significance:

- Did the tests match the data well?

- Are p-values or confidence intervals provided?

How strongly does intervention correlate with outcome?

How accurate is the risk estimate?

Does it make the main finding(s) clear, and do the data back them up?

Does it discuss the result's clinical significance?

Are negative events or their absence mentioned?

Are all pertinent outcomes evaluated?

Was the sample size large enough to find a result that was clinically or socially significant?

Are the results presented in a way that will assist in making decisions about health policy?

Is measurement error present?

Does measurement error play a significant role in bias?

Factors that Confound:

The exposure and the outcome both have a triangular relationship with a confounder. However, it is not connected to the cause. It causes it to show up as though

there is an immediate connection between the openness and the result or it could try and cover an affiliation that would somehow have been available.

6- Which significant potential confounders are taken into account?

-Are potential confounders investigated and taken into account?

-Is confusion a significant factor in bias?

7: What is the study's statistical approach?

-Can participants' primary and secondary outcomes be compared using the described statistical methods?

Evidence-Base practice

-Can I reproduce the analysis if I had access to the raw data? - Are the statistical methods described in sufficient detail?

-Did the tests work well with the data?

-Are p-values or confidence intervals provided?

-Are the results presented in terms of both absolute and relative risk reduction?

p-value interpretation:

The probability that a given outcome would have occurred by chance is referred to as the p-value. A p-value of 0.05 or less is considered statistically significant. We frequently reject the null hypothesis and consider the result to be statistically significant when the p-value is less than the significance level, which is typically 0.05. On the other hand, the null hypothesis is accepted when the p-value is greater than 0.05, indicating that the result is statistically insignificant.

Interval of confidence:

Different reiteration of a similar preliminary wouldn't yield precisely the same outcomes without fail. However, the outcomes would generally fall within a predetermined range. A confidence interval of 95% indicates that there is a 95% probability that the actual effect size will fall within this range.

8. statistics:

-Can the research question be answered by statistical tests?

Are measurable tests performed and examinations made (information looking)?

The reliability of the research paper's conclusions depends on the statistical analysis of the results correctly. The results of the study may be subjected to observational or inferential statistical analysis, depending on the study design and sample selection strategy used.

It is essential to determine whether this is suitable for the study.

-Was the sample size large enough to detect a result that was clinically or socially significant?

-Are the results presented in a way that will assist in making decisions about health policy?

Relevance in medicine:

Clinical significance is distinct from statistical significance as demonstrated by the p-value. Clinical significance evaluates whether treatment effects are real-world worthwhile, whereas statistical significance determines whether treatment effects can be explained by chance. It's possible that even statistically significant minor advancements will not have a significant impact on clinical outcomes. Always keep the following questions in mind:

-Do the results also have clinical significance if they are statistically significant?

-Is the sample size large enough to detect a significant difference or effect if the findings are not statistically significant?

9: In relation to the study question, what conclusions did the authors arrive at?

In the capacity of the study, the conclusions should make sure that the recommendations made are appropriate for the results. Additionally, the study's limitations and their effects on the results should be the primary focus of the authors' discussion.

-Are the research's questions adequately answered?

-Do the data back up the conclusions?

-Do the authors extend their conclusions beyond the data?

- Are the study's flaws addressed and helpful recommendations for future research provided?

-Does the conclusion hold up?

-Bibliography/References:

Do the references follow one of the Committee of Natural Editors' (CBE) standard arrangements?

10- Are ethics taken into consideration?

Was approval from the appropriate institutional or governmental bodies obtained if a study involved human subjects, human tissues, or animals?

-Is the paper ethically acceptable?

-Can you think of any possible ethical problems?

Critical evaluation of RCTs: Things to look out for:

Allocation (stratification, randomization, and confounding factors).

Blinding.

Participants' follow-up (intention to treat)

Collecting data (bias).

Size of the sample (power calculation)

Results are presented (clearly and precisely).

compatibility with the local population.

Evidence-Base practice

Evaluation of systematic reviews critically: try to get a general picture of the results by providing an overview of all primary studies on a topic.

All of the primary studies that were found are critically evaluated in a systematic review, and only the best ones are chosen. A statistical analysis known as a meta-analysis of particular studies' findings may be included. Elements to search for:

Literature search (did it include non-English language studies as well as published and unpublished materials? Did you want to talk to experts in person?).

Study quality control included (type of study; evaluation system for studies; analysis carried out by at least two specialists)

Homogeneity of studies.

Show of results (clear, exact).

compatibility with the local population.

CONCLUSION

Critical appraisal is an essential skill in contemporary practice for determining the value of clinical research and its relevance to the field. This is made possible by a skill set that has been developed over the course of a career. Evidence-based medicine and dentistry can be practiced because they are compatible with clinical experience and the preferences of patients. Such evidence can be considered and applied to clinical practice by following a methodical approach.

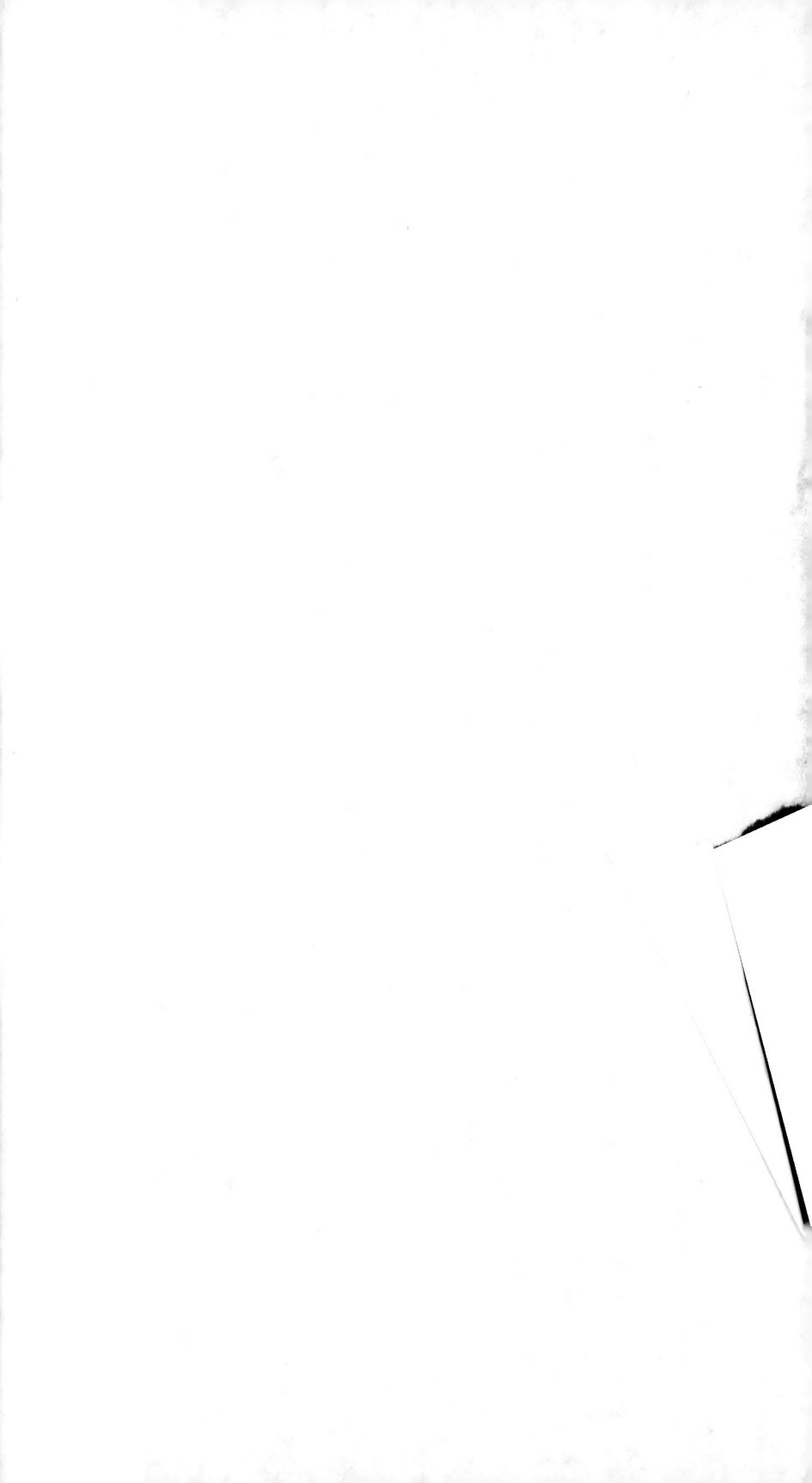

www.ingramcontent.com/pod-product-compliance
Lightning Source LLC
Chambersburg PA
CBHW070302220526
45465CB00004B/1713